Keto Built

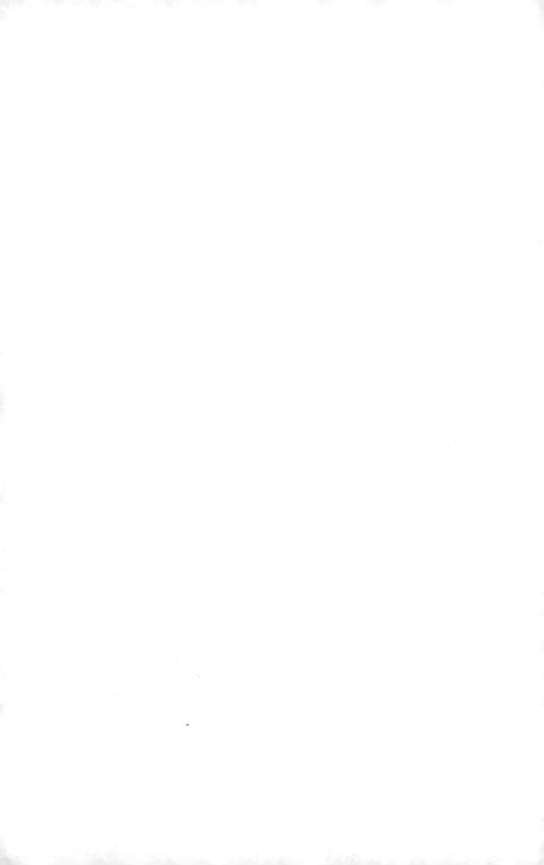

Keto Built

Josh Bryant and Adam benShea

Copyright © 2017 by JoshStrength, LLC and Adam benShea

All rights reserved, including file sharing and the right to reproduce this work, in whole or any part, in any form. All inquiries must be directed to Josh Bryant and Adam benShea and have approval from both authors.

WARNING! Before starting any training program, please consult your doctor or other health care professional. You are agreeing to take full responsibility for any potential risk associated with anything put into practice from this book.

Contents

Introduction   vii

Chapter 1. What Is a Ketogenic Diet?   1
Chapter 2. The Ketogenic Diet for Improving Your Physique   9
Chapter 3. The Ketogenic Diet for Improving Your Performance   15
Chapter 4. Other Variations of the Ketogenic Diet   21
Chapter 5. How to Set Up Your Ketogenic Diet   24
Chapter 6. Frequently Asked Questions   36

Scientific References   42

Introduction

We wrote this book for those of you who are putting in the hours at the gym but are still not feeling sufficiently lean to do your first bodybuilding show, step on stage during amateur night at the local male revue, or drop down to a lower weight division for an upcoming meet.

We have brought you material on weight training, bodyweight training, mental training, interval training, and old-time training. We know a lot about training, and we shared a lot of our knowledge with you. But, as of yet, we had not shared with you the nutritional information necessary to know how to eat and what to eat.

We provided you with the tools to work the part, but now we are giving you the method to look the part.

Using this book, alongside our previous works, will enable you to push some heavy weight, stay #GASSTATIONREADY, and attain athletic success, while also being proud to show off your torso at the local neighborhood tiki-themed pool party.

To find the diet plan to get you beach ready, we looked around for different nutrition options. Unsurprisingly, we found a significant number of possibilities from which to choose. An important element that we considered is the way in which individuals are different in their body types and goals.

If we learned anything from Frank Sinatra (and from many of the "men of honor" who idolized the singer), it is that there is a certain nobility in the willingness to "do it your way." This certainly applies to dieting. You have to find what works for you.

As we searched for diet choices, the keto diet was the choice that kept coming up, and it seemed to offer the best answer to many common diet problems.

As anyone who has attempted to lose those last five pounds before a weekend on the Florida Panhandle or drop some weight for the upcoming alumni game will tell you, dieting is not easy. There are a host of reasons why a diet can be so difficult to start, follow, and maintain.

Often, it can be hard to start a diet because you don't know which one to use. There is either not enough information, or sometimes, in our Internet age, there may be too much information (you may notice that online fad diets are popping up like pills at a Hollywood after-party). In either case, you are left without the necessary knowledge base to choose a diet with any sense of confidence.

Sometimes, it may be hard to follow a diet because of your schedule. Maybe you work long and/or irregular hours, and this makes it difficult to prepare and keep eating the food allowed on your particular nutrition plan.

Once you've been dieting for some time, you may start to get nagging hunger pangs. You might be sitting in class or in a sales convention in Reno, and the loud growling of your stomach draws unwanted attention your way. These hunger pangs can eat away at your resolve to continue your diet.

In this book, we'll cut through the fluff and give you just the right amount of usable information so you'll know how to start a user-friendly keto nutrition program with confidence. We'll also explain the ways in which you can follow this plan with ease, no matter your work or travel schedule. And finally, we'll give you a hunger-quenching plan that will help you maintain your diet without the hunger pangs.

In a most general sense, the keto diet is categorized as a low-carb diet. We found that there are many benefits to a low-carb eating option.

A low-carb diet reduces your appetite. Whether it comes in the form of late-night cravings or lunchtime grumblings, hunger is the worst side effect of dieting. One of the best aspects of the low-carb mode of eating is that it generates a reduction in appetite. The filling nature of protein-rich food results in you feeling more satisfied and, without much of a conscious effort, eating fewer calories.

By default, this diet discourages processed food. The mainstays of this mode of dieting are animal protein and vegetables. Many of the highly processed foods with artificial ingredients, such as flavor-enhanced chips and sugary packaged cakes, are, by default, off-limits with this diet (as a side note, no matter which nutrition plan you follow, we feel that it is not a good idea to consume any "food" that has a shelf life that exceeds your life expectancy).

There is a simplicity to this diet. Specifically, this means that it is easy to figure out what is allowed to be consumed. Once you understand the approved food list, you will have a clear idea about what can be eaten. You don't need to compute elaborate calorie calculations.

Traveling while on this diet is relatively simple. Many diets require meal planning and an elaborate array of Tupperware containers filled with carefully measured food servings. Although the aspiring body-builder may appreciate the visible display of his commitment, the majority of people want no part in lugging around growing stacks of portable food dishes. The foods allowed on this diet may be found at the least health-conscious locations. For instance, even fast-food restaurants offer acceptable options like skinless chicken breasts or hamburger patties.

In recognition of the many benefits attributed to a low-carb diet, in general, and the keto diet, in particular, we wanted to ensure that we included the most up-to-date and easily accessible information, so we reached out to Stefan de Kort. As one of the best personal trainers in the Netherlands, Stefan helps clients achieve their fitness goals through an evidence-based approach to training, nutrition, and lifestyle optimization. Outside of the gym, he is also a prolific writer in the fields of diet and fitness.

Stefan proved to be a valuable resource and provided us with a surplus of scientific information on this topic. We are appreciative of his excellent work.

In this book, we take the research and deliver it to you in the most direct language possible and in a style that is easily digestible.

This book offers instructions and explanations that can be readily understood and followed with ease. However, this is not a shortcut or a magic pill.

As is the case with all of our previous works, this book provides the means and the method for you to get leaner and stronger. You must provide the desire and the discipline.

Chapter 1. What Is a Ketogenic Diet?

On a ketogenic diet, you consume very small amounts of carbs, moderately large amounts of protein, and high amounts of fat. This causes your body to produce *ketone bodies,* an energy source that can be used when the amount of glucose (carbs) in your body is low.

When your body relies on ketone bodies for energy, you are in what is called ketosis, the driving force behind the ketogenic diet.

Sound new? Take a deep breath.

If you have the will, we will show you the way.

We will explain all the important details of the ketogenic diet and how you can work it into your lifestyle. To commence on this journey, here is the backstory on the ketogenic diet.

1.1 Where It All Began

The ketogenic style of eating was first introduced in the 1920s by doctors to treat epilepsy, and it did a great job. Due to the good results, the ketogenic diet gained some popularity among the "lab coats." Scientists began more extensive research into the ketogenic diet, and the use of this low-carb eating style increased as a treatment for epilepsy in hospitals. At this point, it was confined to the lab, not as a tool for leaning out before that summer trip to the Jersey shore.

In due time, the emerging Big Pharma saw the potential to make a whole lot of "dead presidents" with new drug treatments for epilepsy in the 1940s. As a consequence, the ketogenic diet as a treatment declined dramatically. This pushed the eating style almost entirely off the radar.

For years, research on the keto diet almost went the way of the dodo bird, and the masses were almost completely unaware of this style of eating.

This changed when the Atkins diet was introduced in 1972 by physician Dr. Robert C. Atkins. While the Atkins diet was not labeled as a ketogenic diet, most people automatically ended up in a state of ketosis (relax, we'll explain this "state" later) due to the very low carb intake. As a result of the many success stories of the Atkins diet, more research was done on the ketogenic diet, and it led to remarkable discoveries.

Ketogenic diets were found to aid weight and fat loss, decrease the risk of cardiovascular diseases and diabetes, lower inflammation in the body, and improve general health and well-being.

Ketogenic diets were also found to be helpful for the treatment of various diseases, including diabetes, Alzheimer's, Parkinson's, ALS, and even cancer.

It is no wonder that people, in the words of Mark Bell, started to declare their own "war on carbs."

Before you pick up your fork like a battle ax and head off to "war," let's clarify something. Not every low-carb nutritional regimen is a ketogenic diet. There is a difference.

1.2 The Difference between a Low-Carb and a Ketogenic Diet

Even though you limit your carb intake on both a low-carb and a ketogenic diet, there is one big difference: On a standard low-carb diet, your body uses primarily fatty acids (fat) and a smaller proportion of glucose (carbs). On a ketogenic diet, your body uses mainly fatty acids and ketones, not glucose, for fuel. This may sound complicated, so let's explain.

Under "normal" conditions, there are three fuels your body uses: glucose, free fatty acids, and amino acids (proteins). The ratio in which your body burns those energy sources depends on various factors. Those include your activity level, hormonal status, the presence of different enzymes, the amount of glycogen stored in your liver, and, most importantly, your macronutrient intake.

If you consume a relatively high amount of carbs compared to fats, you will burn more glucose than free fatty acids. But if you consume relatively more dietary fat than carbs, you will burn more fatty acids and less glucose.

The same is true with protein. If you consume lots of protein, your body will use more amino acids for energy. (It does so by converting them into glucose through a process called gluconeogenesis.) But if you have a relatively low protein intake, your body will use less amino acid as fuel.

The reason your body fluctuates between energy sources it uses is to maintain stable conditions within the body.

On a "normal" diet, your primary fuel source is glucose. It is the preferred energy source for most of the tissues in your body. In fact, some tissues, including your brain, can't function on free fatty acids. They need a steady supply of glucose (although there is one exception that we'll cover later).

But the thing is, your body can store only a limited amount of carbs. The liver of an average adult male can hold between 100 to 120 grams of glycogen (glucose is stored as glycogen), an amount that is usually depleted after a 12- to 16-hour fast. The average amount of glycogen a man can store in his muscles is around 500 grams [1].

Since you can store only a small amount of carbs, your glycogen stores get depleted quickly when you don't eat carbs. As a result, you have to rely on another energy source. More specifically, that other energy source is ketones, a by-product that is formed in your liver when fat gets broken down.

Okay, you get that there is a difference between "keto" and low carb. But, what in the world is it? On a low-carb diet, you consume enough carbs to meet the glucose needs of your body. On a ketogenic diet, you consume fewer carbs than your body would in normal circumstances need to keep all processes running. As a result, your body produces ketones to fuel bodily tissues that cannot use fat for fuel. When your body gets a vast deal of its energy from ketones, we say that you are in a state of ketosis.

1.3 What's So Special about Ketones and Ketosis?
Remember that under "normal" conditions (normal dietary practices may range from eating fruit as a snack to stuffing yourself with funnel cakes at the county fair), most tissues in your body work on glucose. And while the majority of tissues also can use fat for fuel, there are a few exceptions. The most important one is your brain [2]. Since your brain can not use free fatty acids, it has to rely on another energy source when glucose is scarce—and that is where ketones come in.

The unique thing about ketones is that your body can use them like fats, yet they don't need to be transported through your blood like fats. Instead, ketones are diffused across cell membranes. Because of this, the brain is able to use them as an alternative fuel. In fact, the primary function of ketones is to replace glucose as an energy source for your brain.

In short, ketosis is a state in which your metabolism shifts away from using glucose as the main energy source and toward using fat. As a result, your liver starts producing ketone bodies to fuel various processes in the body.

But besides functioning as a fuel source for your brain, ketones have many more benefits. Many of these advantages benefit your physique. They include aiding in fat and weight loss, increasing your metabolic rate, suppressing appetite, and preventing muscle loss during calorie restriction. The bottom line is that you will look better on the beach and around the pool when you get in a ketogenic state.

1.4 How Do You Get in a Ketogenic State?
Getting into ketosis is simple. All you have to do is consume fewer carbs than needed to meet the energy demands of your body. Under

"normal" conditions, this means you must consume fewer than 100 grams of carbs per day, the amount your brain uses in a "normal" state.

After around 7 to 10 days, your body will adapt to the decreased carb intake. At this point, your body needs less glucose because ketones have taken over a large amount of the energy needs. To stay in ketosis, you need to further drop your carb intake.

The exact amount depends mainly on your bodyweight, but in general, you need to limit your carb intake to between 40 to 60 grams per day. Heavier folks maintain ketosis by consuming fewer than 60 grams of carbs per day. Average-size people should consume fewer than 50 grams of carbs daily, and lighter individuals should keep their carb intake below 40 grams a day.

To keep your daily carb intake in the range of 40 to 60 grams, you should reduce your consumption of, or eliminate, the following foods from your diet: sugar and sugary foods, fruit, grains and starches, alcohol, root vegetables and tubers, beans and legumes, and certain dairy products.

Why is fruit not allowed? Even though fruit contains many vitamins, minerals, and other beneficial compounds, it's rich in carbs. Most people can't stay in ketosis while eating fruit because the sugars found in fruit exceed their maximum daily intake of carbs. However, if you can stay in the range of 40 to 60 grams of carbs a day while eating fruit, then you can add it to your diet.

The following foods are "allowed" on a ketogenic diet: meat, eggs, fish, cheese, butter and cream, nuts and seeds, healthy oils, low-carb veggies, and avocados. You could even eat these foods in massive quantities (without counting a calorie) and the odds are that you will shed massive amounts of fat.

As long as you're creative, there is an endless array of keto-friendly recipes you can make. So, no worries, you can still get your grub on. While you should find a personalized food balance that works best for you, here is an example of how four days of eating can look on a ketogenic diet:

Day 1:
Breakfast: Egg omelet with various vegetables fried in coconut oil, and a handful of almonds
Lunch: Green salad with chicken, feta cheese, and olive oil
Dinner: Pork chops with stewed tomatoes, capers, and rosemary
Snack: Cottage cheese with blueberries

Day 2:
Breakfast: Bacon and eggs
Lunch: Low-carb cream cheese pancakes and a cup of blueberries
Dinner: Pan-fried salmon (cooked in coconut oil) served with vegetables
Snack: Whey protein shake and a handful of pecans

Day 3:
Breakfast: Scrambled eggs with halloumi cheese
Lunch: Mediterranean tuna salad with olive dressing, and a protein shake
Dinner: Pesto chicken casserole with feta cheese and olives
Snack: Grass-fed yogurt with blueberries and a handful of almonds

Day 4:
Breakfast: Eggs and vegetables fried in coconut oil, and a handful of almonds
Lunch: Thai lettuce wraps with ground beef
Dinner: Grilled chicken wings with salsa and vegetables
Snack: 90% dark chocolate and a few slices of cheese

1.5 Exercising to Get Into Ketosis

In addition to making changes to your diet, you can also work out to get into a ketogenic state faster by hitting the pig iron (for you newbies to Jailhouse Strong slang, this means resistance training) in a fashion that depletes your glycogen stores.

You should perform workouts that revolve around high amounts of training volume (reps and sets), with short rest periods in between (e.g., 30 to 60 seconds), and focus on compound exercises like squats, lunges, bench presses, and rows.

Here is what a glycogen-depletion workout can look like:

1. Squats: 3 x 10–12
2. Barbell overhead press: 3 x 10–12
3. Lat pull down: 3 x 10–12
4. Straight leg deadlift: 3 x 12–15
5. Dumbbell bench press: 3 x 12–15
6. Dumbbell row: 3 x 12–15
7. One-leg leg press (both sides): 3 x 12–15
8. Barbell biceps curl 3 x 12–15
9. Dumbbell overhead triceps extension 3 x 12–15
10. Calf raises 3 x 12–15

Exercises in the 10- to 12-rep range are done with 60 seconds rest between sets. Exercises in the 12- to 15-rep range are done with 30 to 40 seconds rest between sets.

High-intensity interval training (HIIT) can also be used to deplete glycogen stores. One example of a glycogen-depleting HIIT workout is 30-second sprints on a (dual-action) exercise bike at 90 percent of maximal intensity alternating with 30 seconds of very slow pedaling (active rest) for a total of 20 to 25 minutes.

For more on interval training, check out our book *Jailhouse Strong: Interval Training*. It explains many of the benefits and applications of interval training. It also includes a myriad of workouts from top trainers.

1.6 How Do You Know If You're in Ketosis?

There are three main ways you can test to see if you're in a ketogenic state. The first one is with a blood test. While this is the most accurate method, it is also the most impractical one.

The second way is with a breath analyzer, a device that measures the amount of acetone in your breath, one of the three ketone bodies [3, 4]. This method is fairly accurate, although less precise than a blood test.

The third way is by measuring the presence of ketones in your urine with a ketone indicator strip (available at most drugstores). This is the cheapest but also the least accurate method.

While you can measure your state of ketosis with the methods above, it is not necessary. Why not? Because ketosis itself is most often not the goal. Instead, ketosis is used as a means to an end, for example, to aid fat loss.

More than likely, you are interested in looking better when you take off your shirt. You probably are not too concerned with what your body is using as its fuel source. Just as with a fine sports car, your goal is for the body to look good, not to have to worry about what type of fuel is in the tank.

So as long as you keep your daily carb intake below 40 to 50 grams, you will stay in ketosis, and you will reap the benefits associated with it. Speaking of benefits, let's look at the effect of a ketogenic diet on your body composition.

Chapter 2. The Ketogenic Diet for Improving Your Physique

By now, you might be thinking, "All this theory about keto is cool, bro, but does it give me a torso that turns heads at the neighborhood pool party and will make this spring break the one to remember?"

The answer is yes! The ketogenic diet is extremely effective for transforming your physique. This is proven by a high number of success stories of trainees on the ketogenic diet, and it is backed up by a fair amount of scientific research.

In this chapter, you'll first discover how a keto eating style affects weight and fat loss. After that, you will learn the influence a ketogenic diet has on your muscle mass.

2.1 The Ketogenic Diet for Fat Loss

The ketogenic diet is an effective strategy for losing fat and keeping it off over the long term. In a meta-analysis (an examination of multiple studies) of 13 randomized controlled trials, researchers concluded that "individuals assigned to a VLCKD [very-low-carbohydrate ketogenic diet] achieve a greater weight loss than those assigned to an LFD [low-fat diet] in the long term; hence, a VLCKD may be an alternative tool against obesity" [1].

Another study compared the effects of weight loss among overweight men and women who either followed a very low-carb diet or a low-fat diet. Throughout the study, both groups were instructed to maintain a calorie deficit of 500 calories per day.

What the researchers found was interesting. Even though the keto group consumed more calories, they lost more body fat and more trunk fat than the low-fat diet group [2].

What's more, in another study, scientists found that even when they had their participants eat as much as they wanted on a ketogenic diet, they lost significantly more weight and fat after three and six months than those who were instructed to maintain a "balanced" diet with a food intake of 450 calories below their baseline [3].

Yes. That's right. The keto group could eat an unlimited amount of high-fat, tasty foods like bacon, eggs, and cheese, and they still lost a lot more weight than those who counted their calories!

Coincidence? Definitely not! There's a lot of scientific evidence (and some real proof from those "in the trenches") that ketogenic diets are superior for losing weight and fat. Multiple randomized, controlled trials show that people on a ketogenic diet lose up to three times more weight than those who follow a high-carb, low-fat diet [4, 5].

Not only does a ketogenic diet offer more fat loss than both a "balanced" and a high-carb diet, research also shows that a greater proportion of that fat comes from the midsection [6].

So whether you want to show off your abs on the Florida Panhandle, drop excess flab to shave some time off your 40 speed, or have a body you are proud to take into summer, the ketogenic diet is your ticket to a ripped physique.

What's more, for most people, there is no need to calorie count on a ketogenic diet. This means no more inputting numbers into your tracking device or weight scale and no more measuring your food with surgical-level precision.

This is bad news for your local neighborhood buffet. You will skip over the carb-heavy, and low-cost, fillers, like potatoes and rice, to focus on the protein-dense, and more expensive, meat and fish dishes. But, to be clear, this is good news for you because you can make as many buffet trips as you desire while staying on your "diet."

You will drop fat and set yourself up to reach your fitness goals as a "side effect" of following a keto eating style. But why do ketogenic diets cause more weight and fat loss?

2.1.1 Why Do Ketogenic Diets Cause More Weight and Fat Loss?

There are five reasons why people usually lose more weight and more fat when they eat keto style.

First off, a ketogenic diet is extremely effective at curbing hunger. Therefore, most people automatically consume fewer calories than they burn. That's why there is usually no need to count calories on a ketogenic diet [7, 8].

Second, a ketogenic diet automatically goes with an increased protein intake. Not only does protein decrease your total calorie intake by being highly satiating, but protein also raises your metabolic rate.

How? Protein has a high thermic value. This means that it uses a relatively high number of calories for your body to digest and process protein. Some researchers even claim that one gram of protein doesn't provide the 4 kilocalories as always thought, but rather only 3.2 kilocalories [9].

Third, a ketogenic diet helps you to maintain steady blood sugar levels. This prevents blood sugar crashes, which means you will experience fewer sugar and food cravings.

Fourth, a ketogenic diet causes water loss. For every gram of glycogen stored in your body, you hold onto three milliliters of water [10]. So if you burn 500 grams of stored glycogen due to a decreased carb intake, you will, at least in theory, drop your weight by 4.4 pounds.

A ketogenic diet also induces water loss because it lowers your insulin level. This causes your kidneys to excrete sodium from your body, which flushes out water [11].

By getting rid of excess water, you'll sport a "harder" and more defined look, and you'll be less bloated. This instantly improves how your body looks.

However, it is important to distinguish the difference between water loss and fat loss. Since water can be gained and lost quickly, it cannot be used to dictate the effectiveness of a diet.

Further, water loss should never be the focus of a diet. While getting rid of water retention improves your physique (which is why many bodybuilders take diuretics before their show), losing too much fluid is detrimental for your health. Fortunately, this isn't something you have to worry about as long as you stay hydrated and you don't use "water pills."

Remember to drink a lot of water every day; sometimes as much as one ounce per pound of bodyweight is warranted. Always stay above a half ounce per pound of bodyweight. This could mean that you increase your water intake while on the ketogenic diet.

Fifth, a ketogenic diet increases fat oxidation [12], so your body will use more fat for energy. That's why a ketogenic diet also prevents muscle loss when calories are restricted—more of the weight you'll lose will come from fat instead of proteins.

2.2 The Ketogenic Diet for Building Muscle

It's often believed that carbs are crucial for building muscle. Many commercial gym trainers, online experts, and social media celebrities claim that since carbs spike insulin, which is an "anabolic" hormone, you must consume carbs if you want to grow optimally.

Fortunately, this is not true. Your body is highly adaptive and is perfectly capable of building muscle on a very low carb intake. As long as you consume enough protein, carbohydrates aren't even required to spike protein synthesis (muscle growth) [13, 14].

In fact, a study of 26 college-aged men with previous strength training experience found that those who followed a ketogenic diet gained almost two times more muscle than those who followed a traditional Western diet after working out for 11 weeks [15]. On average, the keto group gained 4.3 kilograms of muscle. The traditional Western diet group gained only 2.2 kilograms. (Those who followed a ketogenic diet also lost more fat.)

Here's what the study researchers concluded:

"These results indicate that VLCKD [very low carbohydrate ketogenic diets] have more favorable changes in LBM [lean body mass], muscle mass, and body fatness as compared to a traditional Western diet in resistance trained males."

Sounds great, right? So if you want to build a sharp V-shape torso, a well-defined chest, bulging legs that tear at denim seams, and shoulders that take out door jambs, the ketogenic diet is a highly effective option. Here's how to fully optimize muscle growth with a keto eating style.

2.2.1. How to Build Muscle on a Keto Diet

No matter what diet you use, there are three fundamentals you must nail down if you want to optimize muscle growth.

First off, you need to consume a sufficient amount of protein. Protein is the building block of your muscle tissue. This is usually no problem since most keto-approved foods are high in protein. Examples are meat, fish, nuts, and dairy.

Second, you need to consume enough calories. While beginner lifters might be able to grow muscle without an adequate calorie consumption, once you're past the "newbie gains" stage, you need to consume more calories than you burn to build muscle optimally.

To get enough calories, turn to keto-approved foods that are calorie dense, which make it easy for you to satisfy your calorie needs. Examples are nuts, high-fat meat, cheese, and even coconut oil straight from the spoon.

Third, you need to overload your muscles progressively. *Progressive overload* can be defined as the gradual increase of stress placed on the body during training, which allows your muscles to be introduced to new stimuli. This could be done with more weight, increased volume (sets and reps), shorter breaks, or longer rounds.

The idea of progressive overload can be illustrated with the mythic Milo of Croton, a famous wrestler and strongman in Ancient Greece. Milo followed a training regimen characterized by small incremental increases in training weights that added up over weeks, months, and years. The legend goes that as a boy, Milo would carry a calf. With each day, the calf grew a little, and, as a consequence, the weight on young Milo's shoulders would gradually increase. Over a number of years, the small calf grew to a large cow. Milo's strength grew along with it. So, by the time Milo reached manhood, he could easily hoist a cow on his shoulders.

If you set up your ketogenic diet right and you progressively overload your muscles in the gym, those three fundamentals are easily achieved, and you pack on muscle.

Chapter 3. The Ketogenic Diet for Improving Your Performance

While it's still far from mainstream, the ketogenic diet has become more and more popular among athletes. LeBron James, for example, used a keto diet to drop 25 pounds of bodyweight back in 2014. The four-time MVP explained to *Sports Illustrated:* "I had no sugars, no dairy, I had no carbs…All I ate was meat, fish, and veggies. That's it. For 67 straight days."

The ketogenic diet has also experienced a rise in popularity among endurance athletes. There are more and more marathon and triathlon athletes who have finished their races with a keto eating style.

Maybe you heard about the ketogenic diet on a pop podcast or on the social media page of your celebrity crush. Whatever the case, the ketogenic diet is being discussed more frequently.

But what are the effects of a ketogenic diet on your performance? And is the ketogenic diet useful to increase your achievements in your sport? Let's take a closer look.

3.1 The Basics of Energy Production

If you paid attention during biology class, you might remember that your body has three energy systems: the ATP-PC system, the anaerobic glycolysis system (also known as the lactic acid system), and the aerobic system.

The ATP-PC system uses ATP that is stored in your muscles for energy. This system is used for short and intense movements lasting less than 12 seconds. Examples of such activities are short-distance sprinting, jumping, throwing, weightlifting, and powerlifting.

The anaerobic glycolysis system runs on stored glucose. This system operates from a relatively short period (longer than 12 seconds) up to a few minutes. Examples of such activities are a 400-meter sprint, circuit training with 45 seconds on each station and 15 seconds rest between sets, and performing a bench press for 10 reps with a slow eccentric (lowering) phase.

The aerobic energy system uses mainly fats and carbohydrates (for re-synthesizing ATP) to fuel your activities. This system lasts anywhere from a few minutes up to multiple hours. Steady-state cardio falls under this group. The longer your activities, however, the more fatty acids and the less glucose you use for energy.

3.2 The Keto Diet for Weightlifters and Powerlifters

The ketogenic diet has been shown to be very effective for weightlifters and powerlifters. The diet is a godsend for those wanting to move some heavy pig iron explosively while minimizing body fat. As you've already seen, during short-duration activities, you use stored ATP for energy. Thereby, the ratio of your carb-to-fat intake has almost no effect on your performance in those activities, nor does the amount of glucose you've stored in your muscle influence your performance much, if at all [1].

What's more, research also shows that a ketogenic diet produces similar strength and power gains as a regular diet, but you look a heck of a lot better doing it [2].

So why is the ketogenic diet useful for competitive lifting and other endeavors with similar physiological demands? The ketogenic diet optimizes the strength-to-bodyweight ratio because of improved body composition. You will be more effective in acquiring and keeping a low body fat percentage on a ketogenic diet. The bottom line is that with a ketogenic diet people usually maintain more lean muscle mass while decreasing their body fat.

Without sounding like a pop song on repeat, for most athletes a ketogenic diet is the best option. This is particularly relevant for athletes who have weight class restrictions in their sport because it allows one to maintain bodyweight while decreasing body fat. Examples are wrestlers, boxers, MMA fighters, weightlifters, and powerlifters. If you have a lower body fat percentage, you can have more muscle mass while still staying in your weight class. Unless you are super heavyweight, excess body fat can be wasted space!

Another way in which the ketogenic diet can be helpful for weight class restricted athletes is that a low carb intake sheds off water weight. Athletes who have to drop weight often eliminate carbs to stay in their weight class. Then, after their weight has been measured, they re-introduce carbs so that they can compete at a higher body weight.

But the ketogenic diet is adequate for more than just athletes involved in weight class restrictions. Sprinters, jumpers, and other athletes involved in high-intensity, short-duration sports can also benefit from a very low-carb diet.

In those activities, carrying excess body fat will add "dead weight" to the body, which significantly decreases the athlete's performance. That extra weight around your midsection could be better described as an anchor rather than a spare tire, because it's holding you back from becoming the best athletic version of yourself. That's why you won't see an elite sprinter above 8 percent body fat. Most of them are in an even leaner state during their games.

While a ketogenic diet does not directly affect the performance, strength, and power gains of high-intensity, short-duration athletes like weightlifters, powerlifters, and sprinters, such a style of eating can indirectly increase your results by dropping your body fat. This makes it easier to maintain muscle mass and, in the case of a weight class restriction, eliminate water retention.

3.3 The Ketogenic Diet for Combat Sports Athletes

Combat sports like boxing, mixed martial arts, grappling, and wrestling demand a lot from your body. All three energy systems are used during those activities!

Due to the importance of glucose as an energy source in martial arts and combat sports, a ketogenic diet can cause a decrease in performance during these activities, at least during the initial phase of the diet. Trainees often describe it as "hitting the wall" or "the bonk" when their muscle and glucose reserves get depleted during exercise. This condition is characterized by sudden fatigue and a loss of energy.

But does this mean that a ketogenic diet is a terrible approach for combat athletes and other trainees who rely mostly on the anaerobic system? Not necessarily. In fact, when implemented correctly, the ketogenic diet can be used to increase your performance due to two reasons.

First, a ketogenic diet can be highly useful for improving your body composition. This applies in particular to athletes who are involved in weight call restrictions (e.g., combat athletes). By having a lower body fat percentage, you have more "room" available to add muscle to your frame, and therefore, you have a higher strength and performance potential.

Also, as we've already discussed, the ketogenic diet can be used to shed off fluids before your weigh-in.

Second, by following a ketogenic diet, athletes can become fat adapted. This means your glycogen stores will be depleted less quickly throughout the game. As a result, your performance won't drop off as much when a match, fight, or bout progresses. And, remember, you can always "carb up" after the weigh-in, so you can compete at a heavier weight.

We recommend that you give the keto diet and its effects on your weight cut a test run in training, before implementing this in competition.

3.4 The Ketogenic Diet for Endurance Athletes

If you're an endurance athlete, the ketogenic diet is a highly effective way to boost your performance.

As we've already seen, you use the aerobic system primarily during activities like long-distance running and when you do a cardio session in the gym. This system, which lasts anywhere from a few minutes up to multiple hours, uses mainly glucose and fatty acids for fuel.

But the thing is, during endurance activities, it is common that your liver and muscle glycogen reserves are depleted before you finish your race. This can lead you to "hitting the wall." That is, you experience sudden fatigue, a loss of energy, or a significant decrease in performance.

Hitting the wall is very common among endurance athletes. In fact, according to researcher Matt Buman from the Stanford School of Medicine, who surveyed 315 recreational runners, more than 43 percent of the athletes had hit the wall in a recent race. In other words, this condition is the main reason why performance usually decreases at the end of a race. It is also why some athletes fail to complete their races.

Does this mean that a keto style of eating decreases endurance performance?

Yes, this means that your endurance performance might drop when you start following a ketogenic diet. However, after around two weeks, your body will adapt to your lowered carb intake. You become "fat adapted" [3].

Since your ability to burn fat for energy increases, you will need less glycogen to fuel your activities. This shift in metabolism helps you preserve your glycogen stores and prevents you from "hitting the wall" once you get back to a "normal" diet.

To see the power of such an approach, one study looked at the effects of a short-term, high-fat diet on the exercise performance of trained cyclists [4]. For two weeks, the researchers had one group of men follow a high-fat diet. The other subjects maintained a high-carb diet. After 14 days, the subjects had to follow a maintenance diet with a balanced macronutrient intake.

After the two weeks of high-fat or low-fat intake, and 14 days on the maintenance diets, the cyclists were instructed to do various tests What the researchers found was interesting. The time to exhaustion during a moderate-intensity cycling test was almost twofold greater for the high-fat group than the high-carb group.

That's why periods of a low-carb or ketogenic diet can be extremely beneficial for low- to moderate-intensity endurance athletes. When they train themselves to become fat adapted, and then refill their glycogen stores before their competition, they get the best of both worlds. Such an approach is called training low, competing high.

The best way for endurance athletes to use a ketogenic diet is during the off-season. The key here is that you maintain ketosis for at least four weeks. Though your body gets used to burning mainly fat after just one to two weeks, to reap all of the benefits, drop your carb intake for at least four weeks.

At the start of a ketogenic diet, you might experience fatigue earlier and you may notice that your performance is lower. This isn't a problem, and it's just a phase you have to push through. After one to two weeks, your performance will get back to the baseline. Then, once you reintroduce carbs after at least four weeks, you will experience a boost in performance. "Training low, competing high" might be the necessary push to hit a new PR and finally catch the eye of that coed on the treadmill.

Chapter 4. Other Variations of the Ketogenic Diet

Up until this point, we've looked solely at the standard ketogenic diet (SKD). But there is more than one way to skin the ketogenic cat. The two most popular ones are the cyclical ketogenic diet and the targeted ketogenic diet. Both have their pros and cons, and their superiority lies in the application to specific situations.

4.1 Targeted Ketogenic Diet (TKD)

The TKD is similar to the SKD with one notable exception: You consume carbs around your training session. This approach is becoming more and more popular among athletes since it increases workout performance without negatively affecting your ketogenic state.

The main benefit of consuming carbs intra-workout is that it raises your blood glucose levels. This allows for better muscle fiber recruitment and can prevent fatigue. So you will be banging out more reps and piling more weight on the bar.

Consuming carbs post-workout, on the other hand, refills some of the burned glycogen in your muscle tissues. Under normal circumstances, there is no need to refill your glycogen stores after your training, but since your carb intake is minimal on a ketogenic diet, this is beneficial because your glycogen stores will be fairly depleted [1].

But doesn't consuming carbs around your workouts interfere with your ketogenic state? The answer is no [2]. As long as you keep the total amount under control, your ketogenic state will not be negatively affected.

The reason is that those small amounts of carb you consume during your workout will be used for energy. Post-workout carbs, on the other hand, do not interfere with your ketogenic state because working out increases your insulin sensitivity. So the carbs you consume will go to your muscle cells, and your blood sugar levels will drop back to their baseline quickly.

Regarding the number of carbs to consume, get between 30 to 40 grams of carbs after your warm-up or in the first half of your training session. Post-workout, consume another 30 to 40 grams of carbs.

It is best if those carb-calories come from fast-acting sugars such as fresh fruit, dried fruit, or fruit juice.

4.2 Cyclical Ketogenic Diet (CKD)

On a cyclical ketogenic diet (CKD), you maintain a ketogenic eating style most of the week, and you strategically implement periods of a higher-carb intake. One well-known example of this eating style is the Anabolic Diet by Dr. Mauro Di Pasquale. His diet revolves around five very low-carb days followed by two high-carb refeeds.

Alternatively to the 5/2 split, this style of eating can also be done in longer cycles. For example, you might maintain a very low-carb intake for 10 days and then do 2 high-carb refeed days.

The CKD has two main pros compared to the standard ketogenic diet. First off, it gives you a lot more flexibility. While most people find it easy to maintain a keto style of eating throughout the week, it can become a problem during the weekend due to activities like eating and going out with friends and family. Thus, a CKD makes it easier to maintain a keto eating style in the long term.

Second, the CKD allows you to refill your glycogen stores. Glycogen, as we've already seen, is the primary energy source during higher-intensity athletic activities. So, by implementing refeeds before your competition or an important workout session, your performance may increase [3].

There is, however, one large downside of the CKD: You don't get into a deep state of ketosis. Every time that you implement a high-carb refeed, you will interrupt the ketogenic state. Therefore, you don't get the full benefits of a ketogenic diet.

But, as already mentioned, being in a ketogenic state is usually not a goal by itself. It is most often used as a means to an end. Your ultimate goal may be to speed up weight loss, improve health, or increase performance. So is the CKD right for you? Well, it depends on your end goal!

If you're looking to maximize your performance in the gym and you want to have the flexibility to eat carbs, rather than the health benefits ketones provide, the CKD is an excellent choice. The CKD can also be used effectively for losing fat, although it is less efficient than a standard ketogenic diet.

Chapter 5. How to Set Up Your Ketogenic Diet

Now that you have the why of a ketogenic diet, let's look at how we can make it work for you. Here is the step-by-step approach on how to set up a customized ketogenic nutritional plan for you and your individualized goals.

You'll learn how to calculate how many calories you need to consume each day and in what macronutrient ratio (protein, carbs, fat).

Important!
For most people, it is not necessary to count calories on a ketogenic diet. (Only total carb intake must be kept in control.) This is particularly the case if weight loss is your primary goal and/or if you're a beginner or intermediate lifter.

The majority of new trainees (or people who just started lifting the pig iron) automatically drop fat—because they become more effective at burning fat for fuel—while maintaining (or even gaining) muscle as a "side effect" of following a keto eating style.

However, if you are an advanced athlete and want to optimize your ketogenic diet fully, or if your primary goal is gaining weight, we've outlined below the bulletproof way to design your own keto plan.

5.1 Calculate Your Daily Calorie Intake
The first thing we have to do is calculate your daily calorie intake.

To determine your daily caloric intake, you'll first need to decide what your primary goal is. From now on, we will use three situations: lose weight/fat, maintain body weight, and gain weight/muscle.

Note: It is more effective to have one main goal and give that all your attention than to have multiple goals at the same time. The bumper sticker wisdom "If you try to catch two rabbits at the same time, you will catch neither one" comes to mind. It is also reminiscent of the old Texas expression, "You can't ride two horses with one ass." You get the idea.

One common example here is that lifters often try to lose fat and gain muscle at the same time. While this can be done (e.g., in the case of a beginner lifter and by drug use), it is not the most effective approach for the majority of trainees. So decide now what your main goal is and focus on that goal for at least six weeks.

Another important thing to note is that the caloric intake we're about to calculate will not be 100 percent accurate. While it will give you a rough estimation, it might be possible that you have to adjust the numbers a little bit over time. For example, some individuals have a faster metabolism than others, and some people burn more energy in a day due to spontaneous activities like fidgeting, taking the stairs instead of the elevator, and "restlessness activities." This is referred to as NEAT (non-exercise activity thermogenesis).

It is okay if your estimated calorie intake is not completely right, because in general, the numbers tend to be quite accurate. Later, we'll discuss how you can adjust the numbers over time based on your progress.

Step 1: Calculate your basal metabolic rate.
The first step to determine your daily caloric intake is to calculate your basal metabolic rate (BMR). This is the number of calories you would burn on a given day if you did no physical activities.

While there are various ways to calculate your BMR, we'll use one of the two formulas outlined below. If you don't know your lean body mass, use the first formula. If you do know your lean body mass, use the second formula; that one is a bit more accurate.

Formula 1 – Harris-Benedict Formula:
Men (imperial): BMR = 88 + (6.1 x weight in lb) + (12.2 x height in inches) – (5.7 x age in years)
Men (metric): BMR = 88 + (13.4 x weight in kg) + (4.8 x height in cm) – (5.7 x age in years)

Women (imperial): BMR = 448 + (4.2 x weight in lb) + (7.9 x height in inches) – (4.3 x age in years)
Women (metric): BMR = 448 + (9.2 x weight in kg) + (3.1 x height in cm) – (4.3 x age in years)

Example #1 (male – imperial):
BMR = 88 + (6.1 x 180) + (12.2 x 70) – (5.7 x 31) = 1,863 calories per day

Example #2 (female – metric):
BMR = 448 + (9.2 x 61) + (3.1 x 167) – (4.3 x 26) = 1,415 calories per day

Formula 2 – Katch-McArdle Formula:
BMR (imperial – men and women) = 370 + (9.8 x lean mass in lb)
or:
BMR (metric – men and women) = 370 + (21.6 x lean mass in kg)

Example #1 (imperial):
BMR = 370 + (9.8 x 170) = 2,036 calories per day

Example #2 (metric):
BMR = 370 + (21.6 x 54) = 1,536 calories per day

Step 2: Adjust for your activity.
There is a difference in the number of calories a sedentary individual burns and the number burned by someone who has a job with lots of activity or who trains multiple times a week.

That's why it is important to adjust your calorie intake to your activity level. To do so, use the activity multiplier below on your basal metabolic rate (BMR).

Activity multiplier:
- Sedentary (little or no exercise and desk job): BMR x 1.2
- Lightly active (light activity with light exercise or sports 1 to 3 days a week): BMR x 1.375
- Moderately active (moderately active with moderate exercise or sports 3 to 5 days a week): BMR x 1.55
- Very active (very active or hard exercise or sports 6 to 7 days a week): BMR x 1.725
- Extremely active (hard daily exercise or activity and physical work): BMR x 1.9

Example #1 (Lightly active; BMR = 1,900):
1,900 x 1.375 = 2,613 calories per day

Example #2 (Extremely active; BMR = 1,650):
1,650 x 1.9 = 3,135 calories per day

Step 3: Base your calorie target on your goal.
By now, you have an estimate of the number of calories you burn on an average day. The next step is to base your daily caloric intake on your primary goal.

- If your main goal is losing body fat, extract 500 calories.
- If your main goal is gaining mass, add 300 calories.
- If you want to maintain your body weight, keep the same number.

Example #1 (daily calorie expenditure: 2,900; main goal: weight gain):
2,900 + 300 = 3,200 calories per day

Example #2 (daily calorie expenditure: 2,600; main goal: weight loss):
2,600 − 500 = 2,100

Why this difference in range? Fat can be lost at a faster rate than muscle tissue can be gained. A deficit of 500 calories per day is for most individuals the optimal rate to lose fat while minimizing muscle loss. But for the vast majority of trainees, consuming more than an extra 300 calories will cause excess fat gain without faster muscle gains.

Remember, building muscle takes time and patience. While you need a calorie surplus to maximize muscle growth, more calories do not necessarily equal faster muscle growth.

Step 4: Calculate your macronutrient intake.
Now that we know your daily calorie intake, the next step is determining your macronutrient intake—the amount of protein, fat, and carbs to consume each day.

Protein:
Aim to get at least 1 gram of protein per pound of body weight. So if you weigh 180 pounds, you would need to consume 180 grams of protein per day or more.

This is usually no problem on a ketogenic diet since most food sources are rich in protein (e.g., meat, fish, eggs, and dairy). If you do have problems with getting enough protein, supplementing your diet with a protein shake is a good idea.

In regard to protein timing, consume at least 20 grams of protein both before your workout and afterward.

Since every gram of protein contains four grams of calories, you can calculate the number of calories you consume daily from protein by multiplying your protein intake times four.

Carbs:
Keep your carb intake below 100 grams of carbs per day during the initial phase of a ketogenic diet, which lasts around one week, and

thereafter limit your carb intake to a maximum of 40 to 60 grams per day.

As discussed in the targeted ketogenic diet section, you can consume small amounts of carbs intra- and post-workout without affecting your ketogenic state. This will increase your performance, prevent muscle breakdown, and speed up recovery.

So if you're an athlete, feel free to consume between 30 to 40 grams of carbs both during and after your workout. You should not count those toward your total carb intake.

Every gram of carb contains four calories. That means you can consume a maximum of 400 calories from carbs per day during the first 1 to 1.5 weeks of your diet.

After the initial phase of the diet, lower this amount to a maximum of 160 to 240 calories from carbs per day. This means fewer than 40 grams of carbs daily for lighter individuals, fewer than 50 grams of carbs daily for moderate-weight individuals, and fewer than 60 grams of carbs daily for heavier individuals.

Fat:

Now that you have both your daily intake of protein and carbs, the next step is to fill the remaining calories with dietary fat. To do so, sum up the daily number of calories you get from protein and carbs, and subtract that amount from your daily calorie goal. The amount that remains is the total number of calories to consume from dietary fat.

Since every gram of fat contains nine calories, divide that number by nine to see how many grams of fat to eat daily.

Some people find it hard to consume enough fat on a ketogenic diet. If you do, consuming coconut oil can be the solution. Coconut oil offers an extremely healthy fat, and since one tablespoon of coconut oil contains on average 117 calories, it is an easy way to get enough dietary fat and meet your caloric intake.

What's more, coconut oil can even deepen your ketogenic state. The reason is that coconut oil is full of medium-chain triglycerides, a type of fat that gets turned into ketones in your liver.

Step 5: Adjust your diet when necessary.
The calorie intakes calculated above are a rough guess. While the numbers are fairly accurate most at the time, it might be possible that they are not optimal for you—or that you have to change your macros because your body has adapted over time.

How do you know when to change your calorie intake? Our recommendation is straightforward: Don't recalculate or adjust your diet until your progress has stopped over a period of two to three weeks, or if your progress has slowed down significantly. Basically, don't make changes unless there is an actual need to do so.

Regarding fat loss, ideally, you measure your progress based on your body fat percentage. However, since it is not possible for most people to have their body fat percentage tested multiple times per week, a valid alternative is body weight.

What you do is as follows: Measure your weight on the scale every day after you wake up—before your breakfast but after you've been to the toilet if you need to—and write down the number. After each week, add up the days and divide the total by seven. This will give you a weekly average. If there is no decrease in body weight (or below a meaningful ideal rate) for more than three weeks in a row, decrease your weekly calorie intake by 300 calories.

By a *meaningful ideal rate,* we refer to a loss of 0.5 to 1.0 percent body weight per week. So if you weigh 160 pounds, you should lose between 0.8 to 1.6 pounds per week. If you weigh 200 pounds, a meaningful weight loss rate is between 1 to 2 pounds per week.

For weight gain, we will also use the scale for measurement, and what you do is similar. Measure your weight on the scale every day after you wake up—before your breakfast but after you've been to the toilet if you need to—and write down the number. After each week, add up the days and divide the total by seven to get your weekly average. If there is no increase in body weight (or a less than meaningful ideal rate) after a month, increase your weekly calorie intake by 300 calories.

What is a meaningful rate of weight gain? Between 1 to 1.5 percent of body weight for beginner lifters, between 0.5 to 1 percent body weight per week for intermediate lifters, and up to 0.5 percent for advanced lifters.

While it is possible to gain weight faster, it will most likely be paired with excessive fat gain. So if you gain more weight than what is outlined above based on your training level, you might have to reduce your calorie intake.

5.2 Alcohol

One of the most common questions about the ketogenic diet is how alcohol affects the ketogenic state. So, let's get straight to the point: Alcohol by itself does not negatively affect ketosis. In fact, due to the effects alcohol has on the metabolism of your liver, the place where ketones are produced, alcohol can even deepen your ketogenic state.

But, before you schedule a tour of the new local microbrewery, hold your horses.

What you drink has a huge influence on ketosis. Alcoholic beverages high in carbs, like beer, wine, and cocktails, will negatively affect ketosis. Alcoholic drinks very low in or free of carbs, like vodka, whiskey, gin, rum, and tequila, won't affect ketosis. Zero-carb drinks can even deepen it.

However, as we've already mentioned, ketosis by itself is usually not the goal. It is a means to an end. For the vast majority of people, it is a way to aid weight loss.

But let's be honest, even those with full dedication to their fitness goals can find themselves pulled by the temptation to go out for a drink. While alcohol can cheer up most social situations (whether it be a rendezvous with your ex at Red Robin or a weekend sales convention in Orlando), it's also well-known that it can put your physique in the gutter. Also, and not to sound like a "stiff," but heavy drinking can relinquish any chance of "pitching a tent to do a camping trick."

The good news? Your fitness goals don't have to be pushed aside just because you like to grab a drink to ease social anxiety, enhance a class reunion, or unwind from the stresses of life in a cubicle farm. With a little bit of planning in advance and a few simple techniques, you can prevent most of the damage of drinking on a ketogenic diet.

To be clear, we don't recommend drinking to the point where you are wasted, stumbling drunk, attempting to grope coworkers, picking a fight with the bouncer, and making mistakes that could negatively impact your social status and your criminal record. Not only can binge drinking isolate you from some positive people, but it can lead to behavior that is not physically enhancing (for example, a 2 a.m. run to Denny's for the sampler combo and a seemingly bottomless plate of pancakes). Here is how you can have some adult beverages without having your gains go down the drain.

5.2.1 How to Drink without Gaining Fat

While alcohol is often claimed to be fattening, that is not true. The likelihood that alcohol is stored as fat in your body is very low. But don't pick up a six pack of "barley pops," thinking that it will leave you with washboard abs. Alcohol can cause fat gain indirectly. It does so by decreasing the ability of your body to burn fat and by increasing the likelihood that your body stores dietary fat in your fat cells [1].

Therefore, you can do two things to minimize the damage of alcohol. The first one is to lower your calorie intake on the days you drink, so you'll be maintaining a calorie deficit as you head into your drinking escapade. If no excessive calories are floating through your bloodstream, fat is less likely to be stored.

Second, minimize your fat intake on the days you drink. While this will get you out of ketosis, it will prevent excess fat from being stored in your fat cells. So on the days you want to drink, increase your carb and protein consumption.

The reason that you want to make this shift is that carbs only get stored as fat when your glycogen stores spill over. When your liver and muscle glycogen stores are not full, your body will push the carbs (glucose) you consume into your glycogen stores.

Bottom line: If you want to grab a drink with a friend, or alone (we are not judging and we are not therapists), on a ketogenic diet, the best timing to do so is on your high-carb refeed days (if you follow a cyclical ketogenic diet). If you follow a standard or targeted ketogenic diet and you don't want to break ketosis, minimizing your calorie intake on the days you drink will prevent most of the "damage."

But beware. Many people report that they become drunk faster on a keto diet, and that they have worse hangovers when following this eating style.

5.2.2 How to Calculate Calories from Alcohol

In most countries, including the United States, an average drink contains 14 grams of "pure" alcohol. Since one gram of alcohol gives you seven calories, there are typically 98 calories in one alcoholic drink.

Besides those calories, most drinks also contain carbs, which you should calculate as well. To get those numbers, there are various free apps on the market that can provide you with all the information you need.

5.3 Can We Consume Cheat Meals?

Yes. You can add "cheat meals" to your diet without wreaking havoc on your physique. In fact, when done right, cheat meals even help you succeed in reaching your fitness goals. Researchers have found that refeeds:

- Increase leptin, which in turn decreases your appetite and cravings and increases your motivation and libido [2, 3, 4]
- Boost your metabolic rate
- Refill your muscle glycogen stores, which will aid your performance
- Boost your testosterone levels and decrease the "stress hormone" cortisol [5]
- Can help you shed off dieting-induced water retention
- Provide a temporary break, which makes it easier to stick to your diet in the long run

That's right. Whether your goal is losing fat, adding mass to your frame, or improving your performance, when done right, eating stuffed-crust pizza and cheese platters can set you up for reaching your fitness goals. Sounds crazy, right? But it is true.

However, we have to be a bit of a party pooper: A cheat meal is *not* a free ticket to shove everything down your throat that passes your way. If your goal is losing weight, such an approach can undo days of your dedicated fat-loss efforts. And if building muscle is what you're after, the only thing it accomplishes is helping you gain more gut. Both are not the goal behind a "cheat meal."

So from now on, we switch our mind-set from cheat meal to "refeed." A refeed is, in the simplest terms, a planned time frame in which you strategically consume more calories than you normally do. Here's how to approach it.

5.3.1 How to Do a Refeed

First off, you don't *have* to implement a refeed. If you can maintain your diet without refeeds, more power to you. This is especially true if your primary goal is gaining weight. Due to the already increased calorie intake, there is usually both physiologically and psychologically no need to implement a refeed. Therefore, we recommend a refeed frequency of no more than once every 10 days during a "bulking phase."

During a fat-loss phase, on the other hand, most people find it hard to stick to a diet long term when they don't strategically implement a refeed. This can be especially true on a standard ketogenic diet since most people's favorite foods are usually high in carbs. That's why adding a refeed aids you in maintaining your diet in the long run.

What's more, a refeed during a weight-loss phase can also offset some of the calorie-deficit-induced metabolic adaptations. When you decrease your calorie intake for an extended time frame, your body will adapt by reducing your metabolic rate. This means that you burn fewer calories in a day, which is one of the reasons why it becomes harder to drop fat the further you're into your weight-loss phase.

Fortunately, by temporarily spiking your calorie intake, you can (partly) reverse this drop in metabolic rate. That's why—combined with the fact that refeeding makes it easier to maintain your diet—we recommend you do a refeed once every seven days while you're cutting.

When you follow the standard ketogenic diet or when you follow the targeted ketogenic diet, you can implement the refeed on whatever day you prefer (as long as you maintain the frequency outlined above). If you follow a cyclical ketogenic diet, implement the refeed on a day you already have a higher carb intake.

But from which macronutrients do you need to get those calories? That depends on your goal. If you're on a standard ketogenic diet and you want to stay in ketosis, get those extra calories primarily from fat and some extra protein. So increase your total calorie intake through foods like bacon, eggs, cheese, and other high-fat dietary sources.

If you're not worried about staying in ketosis, get the additional calories mainly from carbs, some protein, and low to moderate amounts of fat. You don't have to be anal about the exact macronutrient ratio since you will refeed only sparingly.

As for the amount of food to consume, increase your regular calorie intake by 40 percent. So if you usually eat 2,000 calories, consume 2,800 calories. If you normally don't calculate calories, the easiest approach is to increase your total food intake by 40 percent. (If you refeed on more calorie-dense foods than you usually eat, you have to scale this percentage down a bit.)

You can spread those additional calories out over the day however you prefer. Feel free to experiment to find out what best fits your preferences. Most people, however, find it most satiating to consume them in one meal so they can have a big meal.

Important note: Plan your refeeds in advance. Schedule the exact day and time when you will strategically increase your calorie intake.

Ideally, plan your refeed for after your workout. Since exercising increases your insulin sensitivity, this helps with shuttling all the carbs you eat directly to your muscle and liver glycogen stores.

Chapter 6. Frequently Asked Questions

Q. What happens when you end a ketogenic diet?
When you reintegrate carbs back, you will most likely gain weight. This amount can range from a few to 10 or more pounds. This happens because you'll refill your glycogen stores, which in turn makes you retain water. Remember, every gram of glycogen attracts three milliliters of water. But this is nothing to worry about. It is not fat that you've gained, but water weight.

Athletes often also notice that their performance increases when they introduce carbs back into their diet.

Q. What foods are allowed and what foods are not allowed?
A ketogenic diet does not dictate which foods you can and which foods you can't eat. It only indicates that you have to keep your carb intake below 100 grams during the initial stage of the diet, which takes around 7 to 10 days, and below 60 grams of carbs thereafter.

Therefore, you should reduce your consumption of, or eliminate, the following foods from your diet: sugar and sugary foods, fruit, grains and starches, alcohol, root vegetables and tubers, beans and legumes, and certain dairy products.

The following are foods that are "allowed" on a ketogenic diet:

Meat: Bacon, beef, biltong (jerked meat), chicken, cured meats, duck, game, lamb, offal, pork, sausages, turkey.

Fish/seafood: Anchovies, angel fish, calamari, haddock, hake, mackerel, mahi mahi (dorado), mussels, prawns, salmon, sardines, scallops, squid, trout, tuna, yellowtail.

Eggs: Any kind you like.

Fruit: Berries, coconut, olives.

Veggies: Artichokes, asparagus, broccoli, Brussels sprouts, cabbage, cauliflower, cucumber, eggplant, green beans, kale, lettuce, mushrooms, onions, peppers, pumpkin, radishes, spinach, tomatoes, zucchini.

Drinks: All teas, coffee, sparkling water, water.

Fats: Animal fats, avocado oil, beef tallow, butter, coconut cream, coconut milk, coconut oil, duck fat, extra-virgin olive oil, ghee, heavy cream, lard, macadamia nut oil.

Seeds: Chia seeds, flax seeds, pumpkin seeds, sesame seeds, sunflower seeds.

Nuts: Almonds, Brazil nuts, hazelnuts, macadamia nuts, pecans, pine nuts, walnuts.

Dairy: Blue cheese, butter, cottage cheese, cream, cream cheese, feta cheese, ghee, Greek yogurt, Parmesan cheese, all other high-fat, low-carb cheeses.

As for alcoholic drinks, liquor (vodka, rum, gin, tequila, whiskey, scotch, brandy, and cognac) is your best bet.

You can also include a number of different seasonings.

Q. My breath smells. Why, and what can I do?
This is an often-experienced problem of people who are in ketosis. The reason your breath might get a "fruity" smell is because acetone—one

of the three ketone bodies—is released through your breath when you're in ketosis.

To decrease or eliminate "keto breath," drink enough water, maintain proper oral hygiene, and chew sugar-free gum.

Q. Should there be a difference in the diet plan between men and women?
No. There is no difference between a ketogenic diet for men and for women.

Q. I am pregnant. Is it all right to follow a ketogenic diet?
No. Due to a lack of research, the effects of a ketogenic diet during pregnancy are not known. Until there is more evidence available, we recommend that you not follow a ketogenic diet during pregnancy or when you give birth. Instead, follow a more "balanced" style of eating.

Q. Is the ketogenic diet an option for someone on a tight budget?
A ketogenic diet is generally more expensive than a "normal" diet, so if you're on a very tight budget, it might be hard to eat keto style. However, since most of your calories will come from foods like meat, fish, eggs, oils, dairy, and nuts, you can save lots of money by buying them in bulk.

Q. I've heard ketosis is dangerous. Is this true?
No. Ketosis is perfectly safe. The myth that ketosis is harmful arose because people often mistake ketosis with ketoacidosis. Ketosis is natural and safe, while ketoacidosis is a dangerous metabolic state that occurs only in people with uncontrolled diabetes.

Q. I've heard that the ketogenic diet has health benefits. Is that true?
Yes. That is true. The ketogenic diet has various health benefits. For example, ketogenic diets are found to be helpful for the treatment of various neurological diseases, including epilepsy, Alzheimer's, Parkinson's disease, infantile spasms, and ALS [1, 2, 3, 4, and 5].

Also, as we've already seen, the ketogenic diet is extremely effective for controlling and lowering body weight and fat mass.

Low-carb and ketogenic diets can increase the "good" HDL cholesterol, improve the "bad" LDL cholesterol, decrease blood pressure, and drop blood triglyceride (fat) levels [6, 7, 8, 9, and 10].

What's more, the ketogenic diet is effective at lowering blood sugar and insulin levels and can thereby treat and maybe even reverse type 2 diabetes [11].

Q. Are artificial sweeteners and diet Coke allowed on a ketogenic diet?

There are a lot of different artificial sweeteners, so it is difficult to provide a simple answer. Some of them increase your blood sugar and thereby can lower, or get you out of, ketosis. Others don't increase your blood sugar and are therefore fine on a ketogenic diet.

Examples of sweeteners that do not raise your blood sugar are stevia, inulin, monk fruit, and erythritol. Xylitol is another artificial sweetener that will not break ketosis.

Sucralose, saccharin, and acesulfame potassium are three popular artificial sweeteners that increase blood sugar levels and thereby can hinder your ketogenic state.

Regarding diet soda, as long as the artificial sweeteners found in the drink do not increase your blood sugar levels, it will not negatively affect ketosis. So read the label. Most diet sodas, however, are fine on a ketogenic diet.

Q. Are certain supplements needed on a ketogenic diet?

Supplements are by no means essential. But since a ketogenic diet rules out entire food groups, it is possible to develop vitamin and mineral deficiencies. The following supplements (or supplemental foods) can be beneficial for general health when following a ketogenic diet:

- Vitamin C: A ketogenic diet can go hand in hand with a deficiency in vitamin C. Vitamin C functions as an antioxidant, is

important for the creation of connective tissue, and contributes to a healthy immune system. Supplement with 1,000 to 2,000 milligrams of vitamin C per day.
- Selenium: Selenium is an important antioxidant that fights free radicals in your body. Two ways to make sure you get enough selenium are to consume two or three Brazil nuts daily, or to supplement with 200 micrograms of selenium two or three times per week.
- Sodium: On a low-carb or ketogenic diet, your insulin levels go down, which signals your kidneys to shed excess sodium and water. When your body releases too much sodium, symptoms such as fatigue, headaches, light-headedness, and constipation can occur. That's why it's often necessary to increase sodium intake on a low-carb and ketogenic diet. The optimal amount varies among individuals, but taste is often the best guideline. If you crave salt, increase your sodium intake.
- Magnesium: On a ketogenic diet, you're prone to a magnesium deficiency since grains are the main magnesium source for most people. Symptoms of a magnesium deficiency include muscle cramps, acid reflux, tremors, headaches, and irregular heartbeats. Good dietary sources of magnesium on a ketogenic diet are nuts and nut butter, seaweed, coffee, and chocolate. If you don't consume those foods regularly, or if you're a hard-training athlete, supplementing with 400 milligrams of magnesium chelate can be helpful.
- Fish oil: If you consume fatty fish two or more times per week, there usually is no need to supplement with fish oil. But since most people don't eat oily fish regularly, a fish oil supplement is a great addition to a diet.

Fish oil is beneficial because it contains a high amount of omega-3 fatty acids. Those fats decrease inflammation in your body and help protect you against a number of diseases, including heart disease, autoimmune disease, and mental decline.

Q. What are some alternative nutrition options for someone who has to travel or does not have access to the ideal nutritional options?

If you plan in advance, you can maintain a ketogenic diet in most situations. Examples of ketogenic foods that are easy to take with you when you travel are hard-cooked eggs, nuts, peanuts, and whey protein. Coconut oil can also be used as a "supplement" to provide calories from fat.

Q. Can I eat out without breaking ketosis?

Yes, you can; as long as you keep your carb intake below 60 grams per day, you will not get out of ketosis. So order low-carb foods like meat, fish, veggies, etc. If a part of your dish is high-carb, feel free to ask the waiter or chef to replace it with veggies.

Scientific References

Chapter 1:
1. Acheson, K. J., Schutz, Y., Bessard, T., Anantharaman, K., Flatt, J. P., and Jéquier, E. (1988). Glycogen storage capacity and de novo lipogenesis during massive carbohydrate overfeeding in man. *American Journal of Clinical Nutrition, 48*(2), 240–7.
2. Cahill, G. F., Jr. (1976). Starvation in man. *The Journal of Clinical Endocrinology & Metabolism, 5*(2), 397–415.
3. Spaněl, P., Dryahina, K., Rejšková, A., Chippendale, T. W., and Smith, D. (2011). Breath acetone concentration; biological variability and the influence of diet. *Physiological Measurement, 32*(8), 23–31, doi:10.1088/0967-3334/32/8/N01.
4. Musa-Veloso, K., Likhodii, S. S., and Cunnane, S. C. (2002). Breath acetone is a reliable indicator of ketosis in adults consuming ketogenic meals. *American Journal of Clinical Nutrition, 76*(1), 65–70.

Chapter 2:
1. Bueno, N. B., De Melo, I. S., De oliveira, S. L., and Da Rocha Ataide, T. (2013). Very-low-carbohydrate ketogenic diet v. low-fat diet for long-term weight loss: a meta-analysis of randomised controlled trials. *British Journal of Nutrition, 110*(7), 1178–87, doi:10.1017/S0007114513000548.
2. Volek, J., Sharman, M., Gómez, A., Judelson, D., Rubin, M., Watson, G., ... Kraemer, W. (2004). Comparison of energy-restricted very low-carbohydrate and low-fat diets on weight loss and body composition in overweight men and women. *Nutrition & Metabolism (London), 8;1*(1), 13th ser.

3. Brehm, B. J., Seeley, R. J., Daniels, S. R., and D'Alessio, D. A. (2003). A randomized trial comparing a very low carbohydrate diet and a calorie-restricted low fat diet on body weight and cardiovascular risk factors in healthy women. *Journal of Endocrinology & Metabolism, 88*(4), 1617–23.
4. Samaha, F. F., Iqbal, N., Seshadri, P., Chicano, K. L., Daily, D. A., McGrory, J., ... Stern, L. (2003). A low-carbohydrate as compared with a low-fat diet in severe obesity. *New England Journal of Medicine, 22;348*(21), 2074–81.
5. Sondike, S. B., Copperman, N., and Jacobson, M. S. (2003). Effects of a low-carbohydrate diet on weight loss and cardiovascular risk factor in overweight adolescents. *Journal of Pediatrics, 142*(3), 253–8.
6. Volek, J. (2004). Comparison of energy-restricted very low-carbohydrate and low-fat diets.
7. McClernon, F. J., Yancy, W. S., Jr., Eberstein, J. A., Atkins, R. C., and Westman, E. C. (2007). The effects of a low-carbohydrate ketogenic diet and a low-fat diet on mood, hunger, and other self-reported symptoms. *Obesity, 15*(1), 182–7.
8. Gibson, A. A., Seimon, R. V., Lee, C. M., Ayre, J., Franklin, J., Markovic, T. P., ... Sainsbury, A. (2015). Do ketogenic diets really suppress appetite? A systematic review and meta-analysis. *Obesity, 16*(1), 64–76, doi:10.1111/obr.12230.
9. Livesey, G. (2001). A perspective on food energy standards for nutrition labelling. *British Journal of Nutrition, 85*(3), 271–87.
10. Fernández-Elías, V. E., Ortega, J. F., Nelson, R. K., and Mora-Rodriquez, R. (2015). Relationship between muscle water and glycogen recovery after prolonged exercise in the heat in humans. *European Journal of Applied Physiology, 115*(9), 1919–26, doi:10.1007/s00421-015-3175-z.
11. Tiwari, S., Riazi, S., and Ecelbarger, C. A. (2007). Insulin's impact on renal sodium transport and blood pressure in health, obesity, and diabetes. *American Journal of Physiology – Renal Physiology, 293*(4), F974–84.
12. Paoli, A., Grimaldi, K., Bianco, A., Lodi, A., Cenci, L., and Parmagnani, A. (2012). Medium term effects of a ketogenic diet and a Mediterranean diet on resting energy expenditure and respiratory ratio. *Metabolism, Diet and Disease, 6*(3), 37, doi:10.1186/1753-6561-6-S3-P37.

13. Koopman, R., Beelen, M., Stellingwerff, T., Pennings, B., Saris, W. H., Kies, A. K., ... Van Loon, L. J. (2007). Coingestion of carbohydrate with protein does not further augment postexercise muscle protein synthesis. *American Journal of Physiology – Endocrinology and Metabolism, 293*(3), 833–42.
14. Figueiredo, V. C., and Cameron-Smith, D. (n.d.). Is carbohydrate needed to further stimulate muscle protein synthesis/hypertrophy following resistance exercise? *Journal of the International Society of Sports Nutrition, 25;10*(1), 42nd ser. doi:10.1186/1550-2783-10-42.
15. Rauch, J. T., Silva, J. E., Lowery, R. P., McCleary, S. A., Shields, K. A., Ormes, J. A. ... Wilson, J. M. (2014). The effects of ketogenic dieting on skeletal muscle and fat mass. *Journal of the International Society of Sports Nutrition, 11*(Suppl. 1), 40, doi:10.1186/1550-2783-11-S1-P40.

Chapter 3:
1. Lambert, E. V., Speechly, D. P., Dennis, S. C., and Noakes, T. D. (1994). Enhanced endurance in trained cyclists during moderate intensity exercise following 2 weeks adaptation to a high fat diet. *European Journal of Applied Physiology, 69*(4), 287–93.
2. Proceedings of the Eleventh International Society of Sports Nutrition (ISSN) Conference and Expo. (2014). *Journal of the International Society of Sports Nutrition, 1:11*(1), 1–51.
3. Phinney, S. D., Bistrian, B. R., Evans, W. J., Gervino, E., and Blackburn, G. L. (1983). The human metabolic response to chronic ketosis without caloric restriction: preservation of submaximal exercise capability with reduced carbohydrate oxidation. *Metabolism, 32*(8), 769–76.
4. Lambert, E. V. (1994). Enhanced endurance in trained cyclists.

Chapter 4:
1. Koeslag, J. H., Levanrid, L. I., Lochner, J. D., and Silve, A. A. (1985). Post-exercise ketosis in post-prandial exercise: effect of glucose and alanine ingestion in humans. *Journal of Physiology, 358*, 395–403.
2. Ibid.

3. Burke, L. M. (2010). Fueling strategies to optimize performance: training high or training low? *Scandinavian Journal of Medicine and Science in Sports, 20*(2), 48–58, doi:10.1111/j.1600-0838.2010.01185.x.

Chapter 5:
1. Siler, S. Q., Neese, R. A., and Hellerstein, M. K. (1999). De novo lipogenesis, lipid kinetics, and whole-body lipid balances in humans after acute alcohol consumption. *American Journal of Clinical Nutrition, 70*(5), 928–36.
2. Pratley, R. E., Nicolson, M., Bogardus, C., and Ravussin, E. (1997). Plasma leptin responses to fasting in Pima Indians. *American Journal of Physiology, 273*(3 pt. 1), 644–9.
3. Davis, J. F. (2010). Adipostatic regulation of motivation and emotion. *Discovery Medicine, 9*(48), 462–7.
4. Davis, J. F., Choi, D. L., and Benoit, S. C. (2010). Insulin, leptin and reward. *Trends in Endocrinology & Metabolism, 21*(2), 68–74, doi:10.1016/j.tem.2009.08.004.
5. Forbes, G. B., Brown, M. R., Welle, S. L., and Underwood, L. E. (1989). Hormonal response to overfeeding. *American Journal of Clinical Nutrition, 49*(4), 608–11.

Chapter 6:
1. Kossoff, E. H. (2004). More fat and fewer seizures: dietary therapies for epilepsy. *The Lancet Neurology, 3*(7), 415–20.
2. Henderson, S. T., Vogel, J. L., Barr, L. J., Garvin, F., Joness, J. J., and Costantini, L. C. (2009). Study of the ketogenic agent AC-1202 in mild to moderate Alzheimer's disease: a randomized, double-blind, placebo-controlled, multicenter trial. *Nutrition & Metabolism (London), 10*, 6–31, doi:10.1186/1743-7075-6-31.
3. Cheng, B., Yang, X., An, L., Gao, B., Liu, X., and Liu, S. (2009). Ketogenic diet protects dopaminergic neurons against 6-OHDA neurotoxicity via up-regulating glutathione in a rat model of Parkinson's disease. *Brain Research, 25*(1286), 25–31, doi:10.1016/j.brainres.2009.06.060.

4. You, S. J., Kim, H. D., and Kang, H. C. (2009). Factors influencing the evolution of West syndrome to Lennox-Gastaut syndrome. *Pediatric Neurology, 41*(2), 111–3, doi:10.1016/j.pediatrneurol.2009.03.006.
5. Zhao, Z., Lange, D. J., Voustianiouk, A., MacGrogan, D., Ho, L., Suh, J., ... Wang, J. (2006). A ketogenic diet as a potential novel therapeutic intervention in amyotrophic lateral sclerosis. *BMC Neuroscience, 3*(7), 29.
6. Foster, G. D., Wyatt, H. R., Hill, J. O., McGuckin, B. G., Brill, C., Mohammed, B. S., ... Klein, S. (2003). A randomized trial of a low-carbohydrate diet for obesity. *New England Journal of Medicine, 22*(348), 21st ser., 2082–90.
7. Brinkworth, G. D., Noakes, M., Buckley, J. D., Keogh, J. B., and Clifton, P. M. (2009). Long-term effects of a very-low-carbohydrate weight loss diet compared with an isocaloric low-fat diet after 12 mo. *American Journal of Clinical Nutrition, 90*(1), 23–32, doi:10.3945/ajcn.2008.27326.
8. Wood, R. J., Volek, J. S., Liu, Y., Shachter, N. S., Contois, J. H., and Fernandez, M. L. (2006). Carbohydrate restriction alters lipoprotein metabolism by modifying VLDL, LDL, and HDL subfraction distribution and size in overweight men. *Journal of Nutrition, 136*(2), 384–9.
9. Daly, M. E., Paisey, R., Paisey, R., Millward, B. A., Eccles, C., Williams, K., ... Gale, T. J. (2006). Short-term effects of severe dietary carbohydrate-restriction advice in Type 2 diabetes—a randomized controlled trial. *Diabetic Medicine, 23*(1), 15–20.
10. Aude, Y. W., Agatston, A. S., Lopez-Jimenez, F., Lieberman, E. H., Marie, A., Hansen, M., ... Hennekens, C. H. (2004). The national cholesterol education program diet vs a diet lower in carbohydrates and higher in protein and monounsaturated fat: a randomized trial. *Archives of Internal Medicine, 25*(164), 19th ser., 2141–6.
11. Westman, E. C., Yancy, W. S., Jr., Mavropoulos, J. C., Marguart, M., and McDuffie, J. R. (2008). The effect of a low-carbohydrate, ketogenic diet versus a low-glycemic index diet on glycemic control in type 2 diabetes mellitus. *Nutrition & Metabolism (London), 19*, 5: 35, doi:10.1186/1743-7075-5-36.

CPSIA information can be obtained
at www.ICGtesting.com
Printed in the USA
BVHW030048111218
535315BV00001B/84/P